Your Pet's Health

A natural way to keep your pets healthy and happy.

Complete Guide Book

Copyright © 2016 by Irene Burton

All rights reserved. No part of this publication may be reproduced, distributed, or transmitted in any form or by any means, including photocopying, recording, or other electronic or mechanical methods, without the prior written permission of the author, except in the case of brief quotations embodied in critical reviews and certain other noncommercial uses permitted by copyright law.

Table of Contents

Introduction 5

Chapter 1 – Man's best friend 7

Chapter 2 – Your cat 17

Chapter 3 – Our feathered friends 25

Chapter 4 - Training your pet 28

Final Words 30

Introduction

Your pets are family.

Just like you go to the doctor for check-ups and to stay healthy, your pet likes to stay healthy as well. A healthy pet insures a longer life for your four-legged furry or winged family member. You want them around as long as possible. You want many years of happiness with your family pet.

The problem is you don't want to give them chemicals and hope for the best. You've gone online and been bombarded with site after site of advice, recipes, and information about how to keep them healthy and help them when they are sick, but you're not sure what is helpful and would actually hurt your pet instead.

This book will help you by sorting out the fact from the fiction, and provide you reasons on how the remedies work and what to avoid giving your pet to prevent illness.

You're ready to get to the good stuff.

By purchasing this book, you are well on your way to sorting through the mire of information about keeping your pet healthy naturally. Years of research and experience have led me to write this book. I have sorted through the information on the internet about natural health and your pet, whether you have a cat, dog, bird, or something related to the rodent family.

This will teach you:

How to make remedies for your pet.

What foods and remedies to avoid giving your pet.

Why some foods and remedies can be harmful.

How to protect your pet from parasites, fleas, ticks, and other insects that can harm your pet.

How to apply/give the remedies to your pet.

Are you ready to learn about keeping your pet happy and healthy? Then keep reading my friend. The answers are just a tap away.

Chapter 1 – Man's best friend

Whether large or small, dogs have been a part of many households throughout history. They are the family protector, the nanny, the playmate, and most of all someone who is always happy to see you no matter how long you've been away from home. All stress seems to melt away when you open the door after a long day at the office and see that happy face and their whole hind end wag along with their tail. You want to do what best for them.

No table scraps for Spot...

Unless you make their dog food, you've been told not to feed them from the table. There is a reason for this. The food on the market for your dog is specially formulated to work with their body type and metabolism to keep them fit, lean, and full of energy. You risk a couple of things when you find them table scraps:

Making your dog obese and ill due to certain ingredients in the food.
The way we prepare our food is markedly different from the way theirs is produced. Many of the ingredients can slow their metabolic rate and even make them ill.

They will stop eating the food you buy them.
Constantly feeding your dog table scraps will inevitably lead to them not eating the dog food you've purchased for them.

This means they may not be getting the nutrients they need due to eating the food from the table.

They are at greater risk for obesity.
Since we prepare our food and eat different foods than our trusty pooch, feeding them from our table can make them overweight.

This can lead to health problems down the road, like kidney problems, digestive issues and other illnesses that will have you reaching into your wallet at the vet.

Foods to avoid

There are foods we eat that are toxic to our furry friends. Here is a list of those foods to avoid.

Grapes

This includes their dry counterpart, raisins as well.

They can lead to kidney disorders and irreversible kidney damage.

Onions and Garlic

Yes even garlic, both can lead to increased heart rate and rapid breathing. They can even collapse. Onions can also cause kidney disorders and failure.

Cherries

The pulp around the seed is fine, but the pit and the plant this fruit comes from contains cyanide, enough, that given on a regular basis your dog can die from the pits and eating the plant.

Mushrooms

Only a few types of mushrooms are harmful to dogs, deadly in fact, and if you are not sure of the species of mushroom, it's best to avoid all them for your dog.

If you pooch has ingested a mushroom from the yard, take a sample, and your dog to the vet immediately.

Consumption of this fungus can give your dog seizures, tremors and organ failure.

Currants can cause kidney failure.

Cooked potatoes are fine, but raw potatoes can make them vomit, give them seizures and even cause heart problems.

Apricots are just like cherries. The pulp is fine, but the rest of it is deadly.

Rhubarb can leach the calcium from your dog's bones and cause other severe medical problems.

Apple seeds contain cyanide. See Cherries.

Un-ripened tomatoes and the tomato plants themselves can give our dogs real intestinal problems.

Xylitol can cause seizures and liver failure.

Chocolate has a chemical in it that is poisonous to dogs.

Avocado contains pepsin, which can be poisonous for your dog.

Alcohol is more toxic to dogs than it is to us. It can cause death.

Anything with caffeine can cause rapid breathing and muscle spasms in your dog.

Dogs do not digest dairy well. Some are even completely intolerant. This can cause gastro-intestinal problems for your dog which includes diarrhea.

As little as six Macadamia nuts can be toxic to your dog. Mix it with chocolate and it can be lethal.

Fat from meats can cause pancreatitis in your dog.

Small bones can splinter and puncture the stomach lining or intestines.

Peaches persimmons and plums have seeds which can block the digestive tract. Peach and plum pits contain cyanide.

Cooked eggs are fine. Raw eggs on the other hand, can give your dog food poisoning.

For raw meat, see raw eggs above.

Too much salt in a dog's diet can be toxic. Watch for seizures, excessive thirst, diarrhea, and tremors, just to name a few.

Too much sugar can have the same effect on your dog as it does to you, obesity and possible diabetes.

No raw yeast dough. It can rise in the stomach and block digestion. It can even lead to alcohol poisoning.

Do not give your pouch any medicines prescribed for you or over-the-counter medicines unless it is cleared by the vet.

Wait. I was told garlic was good for animals.

In small doses it can be beneficial. Most holistic veterinarians recommend one clove of garlic per ten pounds of dog and only half a cloves worth for cats, but it's best to consult a holistic vet for a proper dose.

There are many other herbs/cooking spices that are toxic to your family dog. This is also why it is best not to feed them from the table. If you want to make Fido something special, make it without seasonings just to be on the safe side.

There are many nuts we eat which can cause diarrhea in dogs. First and foremost, to keep in mind, your dog is a carnivore at heart. Grains can cause indigestion and an all-vegetable/vegan diet can make them ill. A good dog food will not have any grains in it, but mostly protein from meat sources and some vegetables as well.

Changing your dog's diet can cause them to have some digestive issues for a bit as well, but nothing too serious. If you want to change their food, slowly replace the existing food with the new food by mixing in the new formula with the old. This way, your dog can make the change smoothly with minimal, if any, digestive issues.
Protecting your dog holistically

We all want our dogs to be full of energy, pep, and vigor. We just don't want to have to take them to the vet for shots, deworming, and those pills for heartworms. We want to prevent all that and make the vet wonder what we're doing at our pooch's next check-up.

You need a bath.

Regular bathing can wash many of the germs and things your dog comes in contact with. Its skin, like our own, is your dog's first line of defense against illnesses and infections. Once-a-week bathing is the perfect interval. Bathing your dog everyday can weaken its immune system due to the fact you're depriving him or her of beneficial bacteria as well.

Your dog is social.

Dogs are social creatures. They love other dogs and their people, too. Leaving them all alone in a room can make them lethargic and even depressed. Yes, your dog can suffer depression, and this can compromise their immune system.

Some dogs suffer from separation anxiety, and this anxiety can express itself as a destructive tendency. To avoid this, leaving any kind of noise on, a radio or your television, can allay your dog's feelings of being abandoned. I know you didn't leave them alone for days on end, but they can often think you're not coming back, and lash out.

Beans, potatoes, and dog food

These three things can give your dog the antioxidants it needs to keep its immune system up and running smoothly. Don't give them too many beans. Just like us, it can cause gas. Choosing the right dog food is a matter of weighing your dog, noticing how active your dog is, and then buying the proper food to give them the right supply of nutrients.

It's all about a routine

Just like you, your dog needs a routine to stay happy, healthy, and not be stressed. Regular feeding times and play times are two of the things that need to be structured and routine.

ACK Germs!

You love to take your dog with you to parks, on nature walks and even on vacation. You may even schedule play dates with other dogs at dog parks. These and rest areas have hosted sick and healthy dogs alike. When you get home, don't forget to wash your dog's nose and paws. This will help keep them from getting sick.

Holistic treatments for your dog

There will be many people that say this is not a good idea, but they often overlook the fact dogs can be treated holistically, just like us. Your local pet store has reputable products, but the best way to tell if you're giving your best friend the right remedy, is to ask a holistic vet. There are sources and websites that are hosted by such veterinarians, and they are worth a read.

Chapter 2 – Your cat

Whether Persian, Siamese, or just a mixed breed you rescued from the shelter, when your cat picks you, it's for life, and we all know they pick their owners. They preen, bathe themselves, and can do the goofiest things when they take a mind to, but no matter what mood they are in, they need our love, attentiveness, and our skills of deduction to determine when they are playful and happy or require us to take them to the doctor.

Cats have very different metabolisms than dogs, and thus should be treated differently. They are carnivores, more so than Fido. This means no Vegan diets or veggie-only regimens, unless you want to make them ill. They need meat.

They have modes. This may sound like a video game term, but cats have modes. They have a play mode, a loving mode, a grumpy mode, and a sleepy mode. Once in one of these modes, they can't change them on the drop of a hat. If they want to play, anything that triggers their hunting instincts are at their mercy, whether it be the feather toy you purchased for them or the fringes on your favorite shirt.

On average, cat's sleep eighteen hours a day. This means you're more prone to seeing them napping somewhere during the day. They can be more active at night, which leads to the 3 a.m. rocket races throughout the house.

Just like dogs; however, their digestive systems can't take all the foods we eat on a regular basis. There are some foods that will have you running to the vet because they become very ill upon ingestion and can even die.

Foods to avoid giving your cat

You may think making your cat drunk is funny, but it can cause coma and even death.

Baby food is just that, baby food. It's specially formulated and cooked for babies and can contain ingredients, like onions, that are toxic to them.

No chocolate, coffee or caffeinated beverages. They not only contain caffeine your cat doesn't need, but they also contain compounds that induce vomiting, diarrhea, and are toxic to their nervous system and heart.

Citrus oils can make them vomit.

Dog food, we've all heard it just makes them fat, but in reality, it can cause serious vitamin and mineral deficiencies if fed to them on a regular basis. It can also cause heart disease in your cat.

Fat trimmings from meat can increase the risk of pancreatitis in your cat. So, skip the fat and throw it away instead.

You see them cartoons and some movies chowing down on fish, but repeated feedings of any kind of fish can lead to a thiamine deficiency. This deficiency can lead to seizures and other severs problems for your cat.

Raisins and grapes are highly toxic to cats. They can damage the kidneys.

This should not be said, but any vitamin supplements with iron can cause damage to the digestive system, liver, and kidneys.

Macadamia nuts can damage cat's nervous, muscle, and digestive systems.

Marijuana can cause cats to vomit and can change their heart rate.

We've all seen on television people giving cats milk and cream. Cats are lactose intolerant and ingesting dairy products can cause diarrhea.

Don't let your cats eat garbage. It can cause vomiting.

Skip the mushrooms. It can cause a shock to your cat's system and can even lead to death.

Onions and garlic can lead to anemia in cats.

Persimmon seeds can obstruct the intestines and also cause a gastrointestinal disease.

Raw eggs can lead to biotin absorption problems. It will create an enzyme that will block the ability to absorb biotin.

Raw meat can lead to your cat getting food poisoning.

Rhubarb can lead to digestive, nervous, and urinary problems.

Salt can make your cat have electrolyte imbalances.

Allowing your cats to swallow string can lead to the string being trapped in the digestive system.

Sugary problems can lead to diabetes and obesity in cats.

If you insist on giving your cat table scraps, don't let the scraps be more than 10% of your cat's diet. Our food is not nutritionally balanced for them and can cause health problems for them.

Keep tobacco away from your cat. The nicotine is highly toxic to cats and can lead to death.

Raw dough with yeast can be highly dangerous. It can expand in the digestive tract causing ruptures.

Keeping your cat healthy

Cats can be hard to figure out, but not when it comes to getting sick. It has been proven; most of the illnesses cats' contract is due to a compromised immune system. It would stand to reason to keep their immune systems healthy. Here are a few ways to help your cat's immune system stay strong.

Your cat's diet

Every cat is different, not only in personality and energy level, but also their digestive system. Make sure the food you are giving your cat is balanced to their metabolism and digestive system. It is also best, like the list above, just to avoid giving them dairy of any kind.

Keep them hydrated

Cats will drink water. That isn't disputed, but in order to keep them hydrated between sips, give them canned soft food from time to time.

Hygiene is key

Cats love to groom themselves and stay as clean as possible. You can do your part by keeping on top of the litter box and cleaning it out regularly. There are self-cleaning boxes and even special receptacles for the clumped litter.

Get them up and moving

Cats are active animals, and when they become indoor cats, they lack the activity they need to keep their immune systems healthy and strong. Play with your cats, and buy them things that trigger their innate hunting instinct.

Supplements

Get in contact with a holistic veterinarian to find out which supplements will be beneficial to your cat.

Your cat needs space

If you have more than five cats, you will notice some of them will be lethargic and are more prone to becoming ill. This is because cats need room to roam, be by themselves, and they need room to just be themselves. The less room they have, the less happy they are.

Get to know your cat

Each cat has its own way of doing things and communicating with you, its owner. It chose you for a reason, but beyond that, it's up to you to get to know your cat. Set a routine of feeding times and play times. You may need to change the play times according to when they are more active.

Some cats are lap cats and some are not. Don't be disappointed if your feline companion doesn't like to lie in your lap and hang out with you. It's nothing personal. Some cats will hover and jump into your lap when they want attention and then promptly leave when they've had enough. Forcing them to stay because you aren't finished giving them attention may trigger a defensive response.

To declaw or not to declaw...

This is a hot debate among many cat owners and those who wish to own cats. There are certain things you need to be aware of before you ask your vet to declaw your cat:

Clawing and scratching are part of who they are

It is part of their routine. It's how they maintain their main defense sharp and ready for anything. Giving them things like scratching posts and catnip toys will help steer them in the right direction.

Their claws are their main defense

Yes, they have teeth and can bite, but their claws are their main means of protection. They reach, swat, and grab their prey or attacker with these claws. Declawing them makes them vulnerable to attacks, if they happen to get outside.

It's not just their claw

When a cat is declawed, veterinarians literally take their first knuckle. There is no way just to take the claw and leave the knuckle. This causes them immense pain that does not go away.

Imagine someone getting a limb amputated. You may know someone that's had this done. Ask them how it feels. Declawing a cat isn't much different.

They will behave differently

They may stop using their litter box altogether. This is due to the fact they can't scratch and dig like they used to. The litter in the box is too hard and irritates their paws now. Imagine only being able to wipe your hands with sandpaper. It's pretty much like that.

Chapter 3 – Our feathered friends

Whether small or large, colorful or only one color, there are those of us who love birds. We love to watch them in the wild, and some of us love to have them as pets. From canaries to macaws, there are a wide range of bird to choose from, as well as different needs for each.

Their diet

In order to figure out what type of bird you would like, you have to first know they fall into five categories as far as their diet is concerned:

Florivores eat seeds, fruits, nuts, bark, roots and berries.

Grainivores only eat seeds and grains.

Frugivores mainly eat fruits and flowers, but on occasion eat nuts and seeds.

Omnivores like to eat fruits, nuts, seeds, insects and invertebrates (worms, grubs and the like).

Nectarivores have nectar and pollen as their dietary mainstays, but will, on occasion eat some bugs and seeds.

Even though the seed bag says it's bird food, there still may be nutrients the mixture is missing it may need to be supplemented with other ingredients for a healthy diet for your avian friend.

You can get balanced diets from reputable sources, but you can also check with your vet and online sources as to which fruits and vegetables are good to supplement their diet with to save on the cost of the more expensive bird food.

No, no foods.

Unlike the lists for our other two pets, this one is not as long, but it's always good to ask if you are not sure:

Junk food

Avocado

Chocolate

Alcohol or caffeine

Fruit pits

Persimmons

Table salt

Onions

Apple seeds

Mushrooms

Dry rice

Instead of placing their food in a dish like you would a cat or dog, scatter it in their cage. Birds are foragers, and this provides them with mental stimuli but give them a chance at physical activity as well. You can also use foraging toys.

If you are giving you bird fresh fruits or veggies, the best time to do this would be between 5-6 p.m.

Ask other bird owners and experts on how much you should feed your friend. Too much food will make them sick.

Wash dishes and change the paper out of their cages daily. This will help maintain their health. Always make sure they have fresh, clean water available.

Chapter 4 - Training your pet

This is mainly in regards to dogs. Dogs can be trained to do a myriad of things. There are two main pieces of advice I can give you in training your dog:

Set and follow a routine.

Be consistent.

Think of dogs like kids. Kids learn when you introduce new things, and reinforce them. Dogs are no different. You first need to pick a way to train them.

Snaps and whistles

Any short loud sound will get their attention. Following it up by issuing a command will teach them what to do according to the sound, duration of the sound, and how many times you repeat it.

For instance, to get them to sit, snap your fingers once while telling them to sit and pushing down on their backside. This will teach them to sit to the point where all you will have to do is snap and utter the command.

Verbal Commands

This is like the above method, just without the noise.

Housebreaking

This can be a challenge, especially if you are away from the house for work. Get them into the habit of going outside about an hour after you feed them by taking them outside to do their business. If they are small dogs, you can train them to use puppy pads indoors.

Crate training

I don't endorse this type of training, but if you have a dog that exhibits destructive tendencies you can't seem to train out of them, this may be the only to keep your place in one piece and your pet safe.

Final Words

We all want happy and healthy pets. In order to have that, we have to do what is right. Make sure you've done your homework in regards to the pet you are looking to acquire.

A pet is a life-time commitment, at least for the pet. You are their family now, and they are your responsibility. Make sure you are ready to own a pet. You can do this by making sure:

You have a home suitable for raising and caring for an animal;

You can spend time bonding and playing with your pet;

You are able to keep up with the demands of keeping them and their areas clean; and

You are fully committed to meeting their needs.

There are plenty of online sources which can help you and forums you can be a part of so you can talk to and get tips and advice on how to care for your pet.

www.ingramcontent.com/pod-product-compliance
Lightning Source LLC
Chambersburg PA
CBHW061238180526
45170CB00003B/1358